Ch

Coupons

Happy Christmas

Copyright © 2016 Happy Christmas

All rights reserved.

ISBN:10: 1540851273
ISBN-13: 978-1540851277

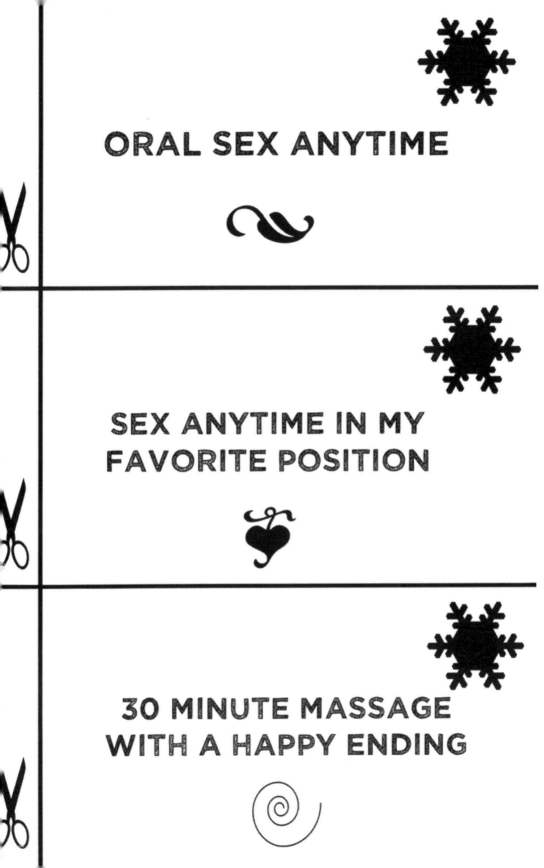

Backside of Coupon

Backside of Coupon

Backside of Coupon

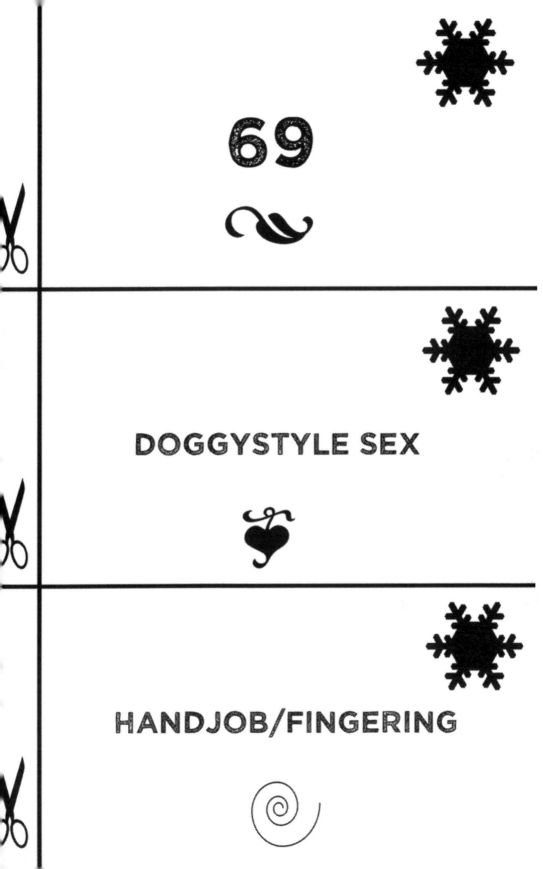

Backside of Coupon

Backside of Coupon

Backside of Coupon

REVERSE 69

MISSIONARY SEX

TIE YOU UP AND HAVE MY WAY WITH YOU FOR A NIGHT

Backside of Coupon

Backside of Coupon

Backside of Coupon

SIDEWAYS 69

COWGIRL SEX

BUY A SEX TOY AND WE USE IT LATER THIS WEEK

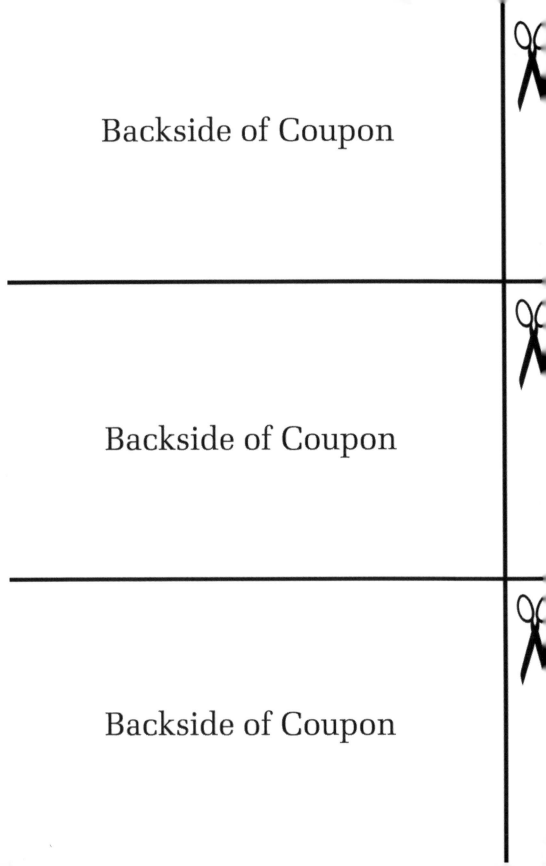

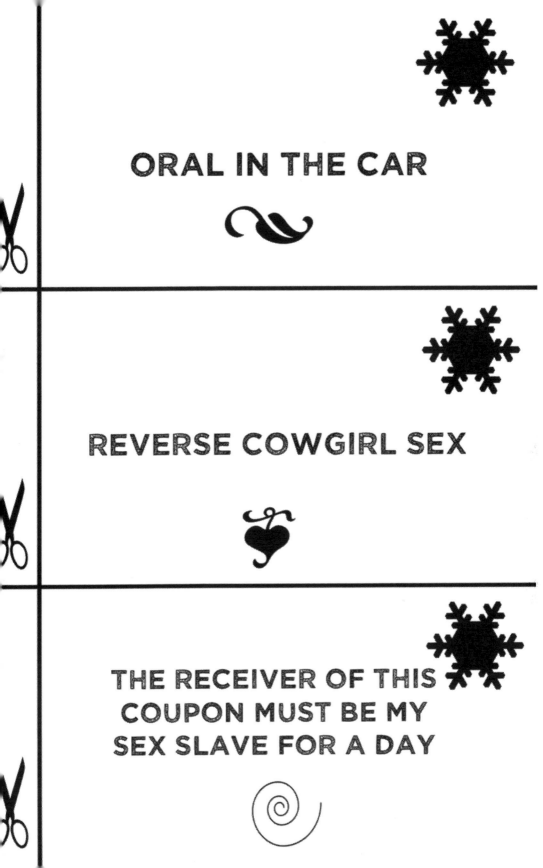

Backside of Coupon

Backside of Coupon

Backside of Coupon

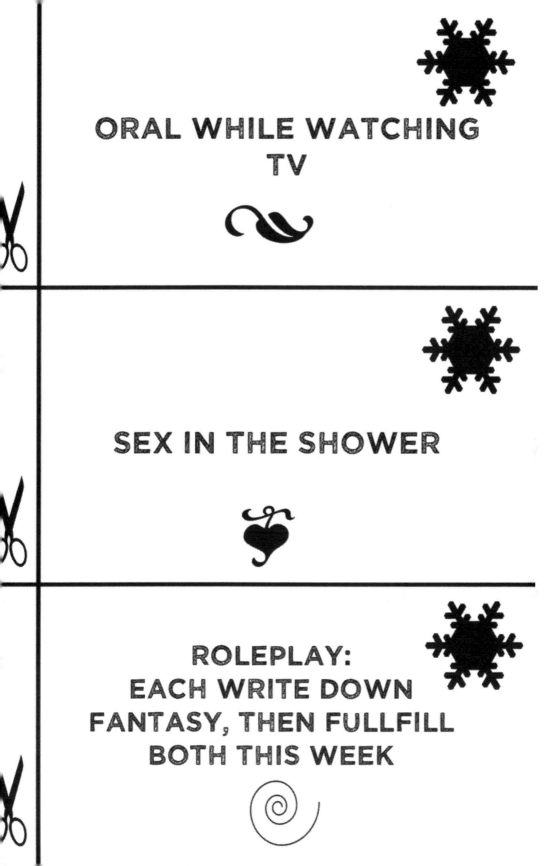

Backside of Coupon

Backside of Coupon

Backside of Coupon

MAKE ME BREAKFAST
IN BED AND WHILE I EAT
GIVE ME ORAL LOVE

DIRTY KITCHEN SEX
CHOCOLATE SYRUP
AND WHIP CREAM OPTIONAL

MORNING SEX
NO QUESTIONS ASKED

Backside of Coupon

Backside of Coupon

Backside of Coupon

STRIP TEASE SHOW

NAKED YOGA SEX
HOW MANY YOGA POSITIONS DO YOU KNOW?

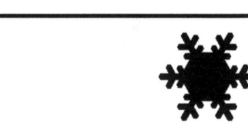

ONE QUICKIE

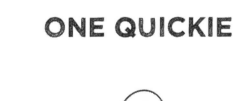

Backside of Coupon

Backside of Coupon

Backside of Coupon

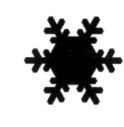

**PUT ON A SEXY OUTFIT
SEX**

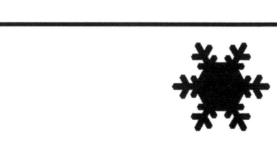

**GO OUT WITH NO UNDERWEAR
AND FILL ME UP UNDER THE TABLE
HOW FAR WILL IT GO?**

**FINGER MY BUTT, WHILE
YOU DO ME FROM BEHIND
SEX**

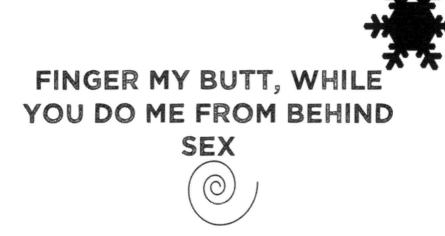

Backside of Coupon

Backside of Coupon

Backside of Coupon

ORAL IN THE BATHTUB

SEX SOMEWHERE WE HAVE NEVER DONE IT.

TAKE ME OUT TO DINNER AND TOUCH ME, KISS ME, AND FONDLE ME.

Backside of Coupon

Backside of Coupon

Backside of Coupon

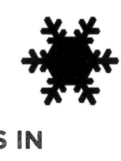

MAKE ME CUM 3 TIMES IN A DAY

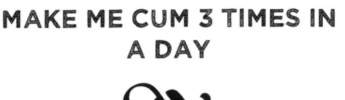

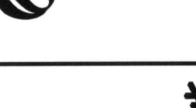

ORAL WHILE I AM SLEEPING, WAKE ME UP.

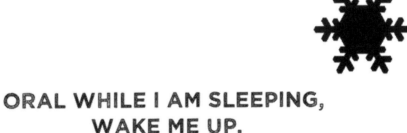

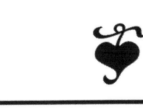

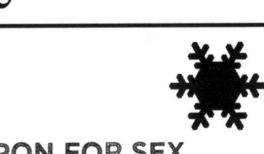

FREE COUPON FOR SEX IN THE MIDDLE OF THE NIGHT

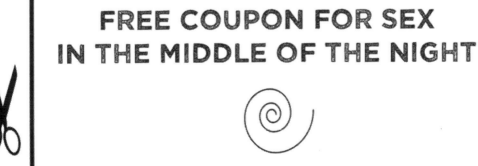

Backside of Coupon

Backside of Coupon

Backside of Coupon

MY FAVORITE SEX POSITION

YOUR FAVORITE SEX POSITION

SEX IN A COSTUME ROLEPLAY

Backside of Coupon

Backside of Coupon

Backside of Coupon

Made in the USA
Columbia, SC
05 December 2018